Health and Fitness Mindset for Life

Change the Way You Think to Implement Healthy Lifestyle Changes that Will Last

Kelly Larson

This book is dedicated to anyone who is ready to change their mindset and choose overall wellness over excuses, fad diets and fitness programs. Change your outlook and you can change your life.

Copyright Act of 1976, the scanning, uploading and electronic sharing of any part of this book without the explicit written consent or permission of the publisher constitutes unlawful piracy and the theft of intellectual property.

If you would like to use material or content from this book (other than for review purposes), prior written permission must be obtained from the publisher.

You can contact the publishing company at admin@speedypublishing.com. Thank you for not infringing on the author's rights.

Speedy Publishing LLC (c) 2014
40 E. Main St., #1156
Newark, DE 19711
www.speedypublishing.co

Ordering Information:
Quantity sales; Special discounts are available on quantity purchases by corporations, associations, and others. For details, contact the "Special Sales Department" at the address above.

This is a reprint book.

Manufactured in the United States of America

Table of Contents

Publisher's Notes i

Introduction 1

Chapter 1: Why Do New Health and Fitness Goals Result in Failure? 2

Chapter 2: How Will You Stay Motivated? 4

Chapter 3: How to Select the Right Program for You 6

Chapter 4: Start Out Slow 9

Chapter 5: Targeting Your Body's Problem Areas 11

Chapter 6: Get Your Friends or Family Involved 14

Chapter 7: Track Your Progress 16

Chapter 8: Stay Motivated with Incentives 18

Chapter 9: Make the Effort – Exercise Even if You Don't Feel Like It 20

Chapter 10: You Can Do It! Sticking to Your Health and Fitness Goals 22

Chapter 11: Health and Fitness Affirmations 24

Meet the Author 33

More Books by Kelly Larson 34

Publisher's Notes

Disclaimer

This publication is intended to provide helpful and informative material. It is not intended to diagnose, treat, cure, or prevent any health problem or condition, nor is intended to replace the advice of a physician. No action should be taken solely on the contents of this book. Always consult your physician or qualified health-care professional on any matters regarding your health and before adopting any suggestions in this book or drawing inferences from it.

The author and publisher specifically disclaim all responsibility for any liability, loss or risk, personal or otherwise, which is incurred as a consequence, directly or indirectly, from the use or application of any contents of this book.

Any and all product names referenced within this book are the trademarks of their respective owners. None of these owners have sponsored, authorized, endorsed, or approved this book.

Always read all information provided by the manufacturers' product labels before using their products. The author and publisher are not responsible for claims made by manufacturers.

INTRODUCTION

It happens over and over again – we resolve to start a health and fitness program with gusto and probably much fanfare too. This time we are going to stick to it. But within the first month or even first week, we lose our motivation and our goals and dreams fizzle out yet again.

Why is it that we don't stick to the diet plans, the morning jog, the workout plans that we make?

And what can we do to ensure we stick to these plans, for our own sake and for the sake of the people that are dependent on us?

Chapter 1: Why Do New Health and Fitness Goals Result in Failure?

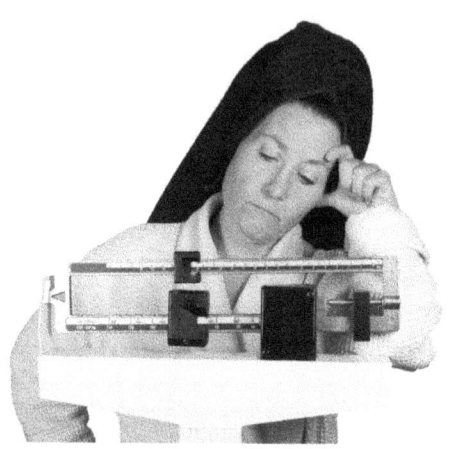

In today's world, rarely do health and fitness programs work. What's the reason for their alarming rate of failure?

Why Do Most Health and Fitness Programs Fail?

We hear it a lot – Someone takes a gym membership and then lets it die without a whimper. Someone takes up a diet and then returns to gluttony the next weekend. Someone does a great deal of expensive shopping from big-name brands for morning routines and then wears the filthily expensive tracksuit for lounging around at home. This bug is all around us – People make grandiose plans to start health and fitness programs and then let go of them at the drop of a hat. What goes wrong?

When we hear about the failure of diets or gym programs all around us, usually it isn't their fault. Usually it is the fault of the people who started with much hoo-ha about going through these programs, telling all their friends and colleagues about it, and then did not follow those programs through to the end. The people who leave midway do not see the benefits, of course, and the commercial fitness enterprises lose their face.

What the world needs today isn't a new health or fitness program, but it needs motivation. It needs the right kind of mindset to follow through with whatever program they have chosen to the very end. If they can do that, most of the health problems that are related to lifestyle situations will become passé. And we don't have to travel to the corners of the earth to find this motivation. The motivation lies right here, within us; we only need to search it and use it.

And this we need to do before even thinking of joining a health program.

So the next time you see that a program has failed or is receiving a lot of criticism, remember that the criticism isn't probably because the program stands on shaky ground. In most cases, it is because people began with great intentions and then did not follow the program as they should have.

Chapter 2: How Will You Stay Motivated?

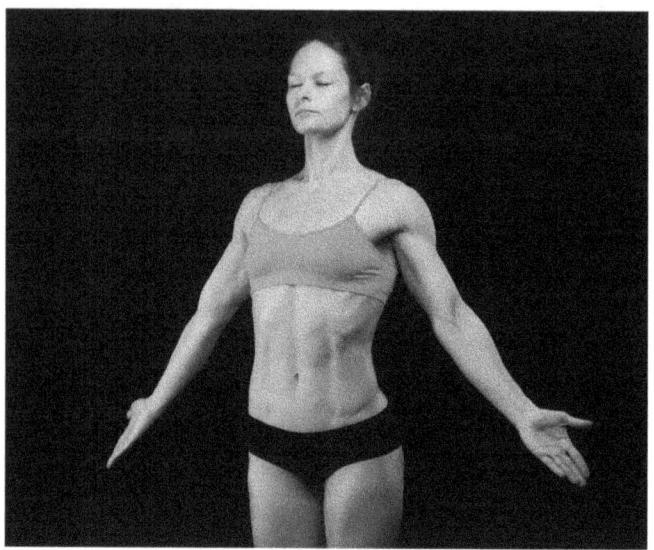

The main thing you need is motivation. As it is true in everything in life that you do, it is true here as well.

Determination and Motivation – Your Most Important Allies

The most important thing that you need to keep your health and fitness program alive – even more important than an instructor or a doctor – is your own motivation. You have to be determined to take stock of the situation. So, you are overweight and are looking at shedding some pounds. No gym instructor from anywhere in the world will help you if you don't take adequate measures to have the right diet and to stick with your routine exercise. Even if you are sick and are looking at treatment, no doctor will help if you aren't determined in following the treatment program, whether it is taking the medication at the right time or abstaining from some foods.

Even God can't help people who don't help themselves.

So, before even thinking of going ahead with a fitness or a health program, the one thing you need to be sure of is your own determination for it.

You have to make sure you will be motivated to carry on the program till the end. The best way to do it, of course, is to think about the end result. If you are planning to enter into a weight loss program, you could think about the great body you will have if you follow the program for a few weeks. In fact, you could go right ahead and shop for some jeans or even a bikini which is five sizes smaller than you are presently. The people who sell you that will think you are nuts, but you know what you are trying to achieve. Actually, stand up and tell them that this is what size you will be when you enter their shop again!

The same applies for every health and fitness program. If you have some cardiac ailment right now, think about how sticking to the right medical program will make you feel after a few weeks. You will be able to do things as before; your life will be richer.

The best way to keep yourself motivated is always to think about what is to come. Think about the result of your efforts. The efforts you need to put in won't seem so very difficult then.

Chapter 3: How to Select the Right Program for You

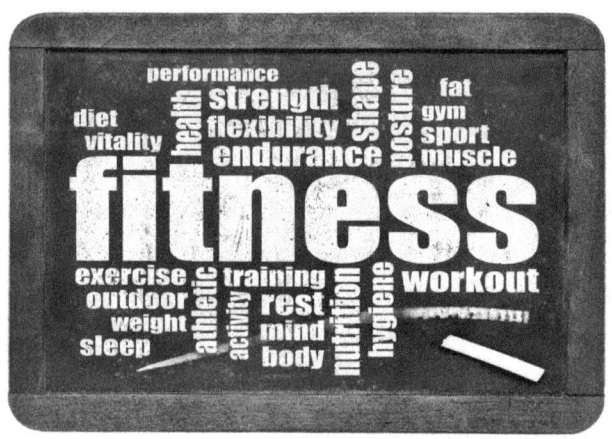

It is highly important to choose the right program from the crowd.

Selecting the Right Program

The health and fitness industry is probably the most saturated industry in the world today. Part of the reason for that is people try out one program and then fail because of their own lack of determination and then think the program is worthless and try another. What the health and fitness industry doesn't tell people on their face is that they are failing mostly because they are not able to resolve themselves to stick to one program. They will probably fail with this one too because their minds are rolling stones, but it doesn't matter because presently they are spending thousands of dollars on buying their products.

It works that way. But the fact is that the industry is saturated. So what do you do when you are looking at a program for yourself? If it is a health treatment program, your choice is simpler. You just go to a doctor that you have faith in – usually your family physician – and then do as they say. But the issue is very much complicated if you are looking for a viable fitness program. What do you use to stay fit – diet, exercise, aerobics, calisthenics, what?

Researching on the Internet is not the answer. What you will find mostly is articles full of sales pitch, written by people who are trying to promote their own product. They won't have any qualms in painting some other perfectly good product with a negative color if they can improve the impression of their own product. The world gobbles it up, so it works.

Now, if you want to choose a program, the best thing you could do is to head to your nearest bookstore. You should first narrow your choices to two or three fitness programs that really interest you. It is great if you can speak to some people who have used the programs you are contemplating and who have absolutely no commercial interests whatsoever in promoting what they are doing. Join a health and fitness club. This is a great place to meet people who are conscious about their fitness and they won't mind giving you great advice.

When you get the material on what programs you are thinking about, take the time to read them. Read them mainly to understand what you will have to do, how much time you will have to devote, what equipment you will need, whether you will be able to do what is mentioned, what the results will be and how soon you will get them, etc. These facts will help you decide whether you want to commit to the program.

Don't trust anybody when it comes to deciding a fitness program for you. Most people will have commercial interests. Some well-meaning souls will give you advice too, but they may be limited in their knowledge. It is best to speak with impartial experts, like your doctor, do your own research form an initial decision. Of course, you need to speak with a qualified person before making your eventual decision about what program will be best for you.

CHAPTER 4: START OUT SLOW

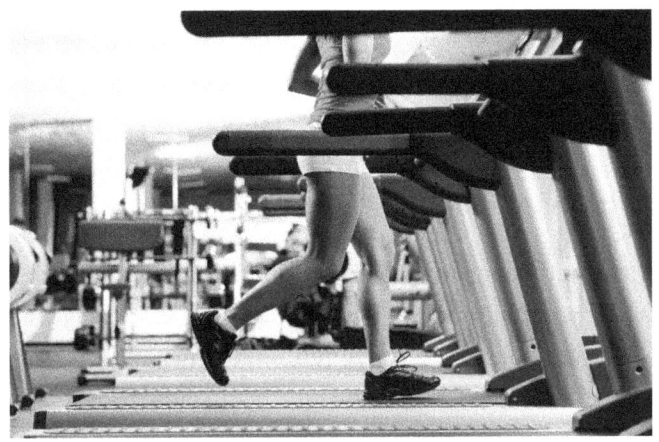

Fools rush in; wise men take things one day at a time.

Starting Slow

The key is to start slow. When you start your health and fitness program at a slow pace, you will be more comfortable and ease yourself into new habits.

So, when you embarking on your fitness regimen, don't rush in and overdo it. For example, if you are going to jog each morning, don't plan on jogging for an hour on your first day. Start slow – maybe do just ten to fifteen minutes the first day. You may not have exercised in a long time. Hence, you will be activating muscles and body parts that have been idle. Also consider you will need to build up your stamina to be able to exert yourself for longer periods of time. If you go all out on your first day you will be exhausted and sore and may be unable to physically exercise for a few days until your body recovers. Will you still be motivated to restart your fitness regimen?

The same applies when you are going to change your eating habits. If you drastically change your eating habits without the proper mindset you may feel mental and physical withdrawal symptoms from eliminating sugar, carbohydrates, caffeine, etc. and fall into depression which can make you give up quickly. Depression also does something that will be detrimental to your weight loss plan. It releases a hormone known as cortisol. This hormone, also known as the stress hormone, will make you mentally weak and will make you vulnerable. You will give up your plan sooner because of the release of this hormone.

Instead, start off by giving up a few of the unhealthy items at the beginning of your new regime and work on eliminating unhealthy fats, sugars, and processed carbohydrates over the period of a few weeks to a month. Even though you are trying to eat clean and healthy, it is okay to indulge one interesting meal per week so that you don't feel deprived. If you have a day that you blow your eating plan, do not beat yourself up with negative self-talk and become derailed from your goals. Bad days will happen and while it is useful to understand why you choose to eat poorly(emotions, lack of planning, portion control, availability of tempting food, etc.) you need to let it go and move forward. It is important to remember that the next day is a new day with a clean slate.

Reduction is a successful approach for many people who are trying to give up smoking They begin cutting down on the number of cigarettes they smoke each day. Over time, they drastically reduce their extent of smoking. This method can be applied to food and diet as well.

When you are starting a long-term health and fitness plan, it is best to start slow and build momentum with small successful baby steps. This builds a strong foundation for long term health and fitness changes.

Chapter 5: Targeting Your Body's Problem Areas

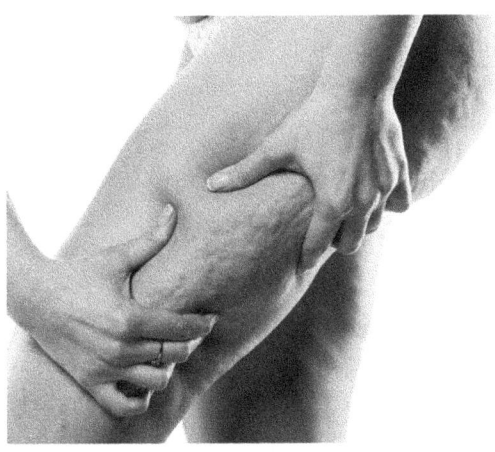

Specialization and prioritization are two essentials if you want to do things the most efficient way, especially when it comes to deciding a suitable health and fitness plan for your needs.

Target the Right Parts of the Body

One of the biggest problems in following health and fitness programs arise when people don't know and understand what they should really do. Being uninformed or misinformed can lead to exercise that is ineffective. This leads to time spent and physical exertion that does not produce desired results. This then leads to frustration which can unmotivated many.

Take the example of someone who wants to shape, define and increase strength in their legs. If this person solely focuses on upper body exercises they will be disappointed with the lack of results in their legs. This is a simple example but the point is to set goals and do your homework on researching what methods will bring the results you desire.

Fitness magazines are an excellent resource and are targeted for both men and women. Thumb through and find someone who has the abs, arms, legs, etc. that YOU want. Their workout routines are often listed. Tear out the pages with their picture (for motivation) and their routine. You can do this for each area of your body that you want to improve. This ensures you are doing the correct exercises for your specific problem areas. Just remember to start out with fewer reps and lighter weights and increase gradually over time.

Some people prioritize their fitness regimens. They decide what they want to focus on first and direct their time and energy on that problem area. When that aspect of their fitness has improved, they move on to the next problem area. Such focused attention works quite well, especially in today's world where we are all cramped for time and don't want to spare the effort either.

That is why most gyms have various structured programs for working out. If you are joining a gym after a long time of physical inactivity, you may find that they will instruct you to focus more on building up your stamina. For that, you will probably find yourself on cardio equipment such as the treadmill or an exercise bike a lot initially. Once you have built up some stamina you will slowly start working resistance training into your fitness routine.

If you ignore the advice of starting slow and go all out on your first day, or first week, you will stress your body. There is potential for strains, tears, and injuries setting you back which could be disastrous to your long-term goals and your motivation. In the very least, by pushing yourself too hard in the beginning you might find yourself sore and barely able to move throughout your normal day. When that happens, people don't stick to their fitness plans and goals.

The mistake here isn't of the program itself; it is of the way in which you approached it.

CHAPTER 6: GET YOUR FRIENDS OR FAMILY INVOLVED

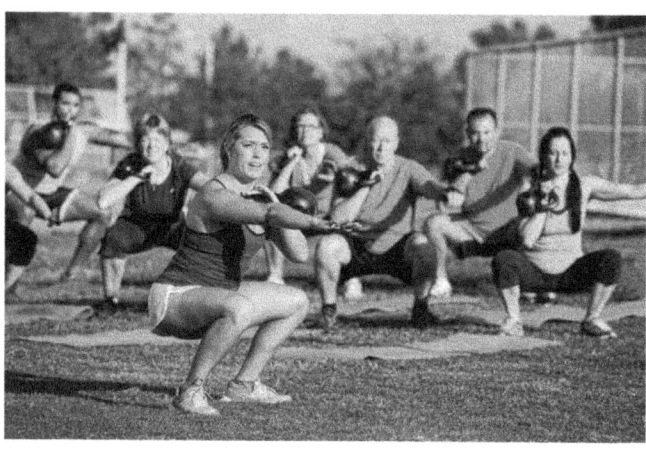

Friends and family can be helpful when you are starting or maintaining a health and fitness program. They could be the support system you need to stay motivated and hold you accountable.

Your friends or family could be very instrumental in making you stick with your fitness goals. Many health and fitness advocates say that people who work out with a friend or fitness partner, are more likely to achieve their goals. If you have someone to go to the gym with you, or diet with you, or accompany you on your morning jogs, you will be more apt to stick to your routine and to the program itself.

There are many reasons why it works. The main reason is that the boredom does not creep in when you have a friend or partner to work out with. We aren't as likely to be bored when we are around others, are we? Also, a healthy competition triggered between the two of you is beneficial in pushing both of you to do better. You might want to see who can lift more, who can jog further, who can lose more weight, etc. All this keeps you focused on your fitness goals and also keeps you motivated.

But if you cannot find a friend or family member to work out with you, you can involve them in other constructive ways. Tell the world you are making healthy lifestyle change in diet and/or fitness. Hopefully they will be supportive and encourage you. But, what if they don't support you and are negative? They roll their eyes and tell you that you'll never be able to stick it out? Use their doubt and negativity to motivate you to prove them wrong. Take their negativity personally and turn it into a positive thing. Use their fears and doubts to stay focused and work harder. Negative people can ignite a fire in you and keep you motivated even when they don't know that's what they are doing.

The next time you are with a friend who knows you have health and fitness goals and are tempted to gorge on something with no nutritional value, you will think twice about it. Chances are you will pass and won't eat it. Instead you will make a smart and healthy decision. That is because you don't want to falsify your resolve in front of a friend. But if you haven't told your friend about your lifestyle changes, you might have no qualms about binging with them.

This is how friends and family help you. Even if they don't say anything, and are unlikely to do so, you know they know and this helps you stay on track with your health and fitness goals.

CHAPTER 7: TRACK YOUR PROGRESS

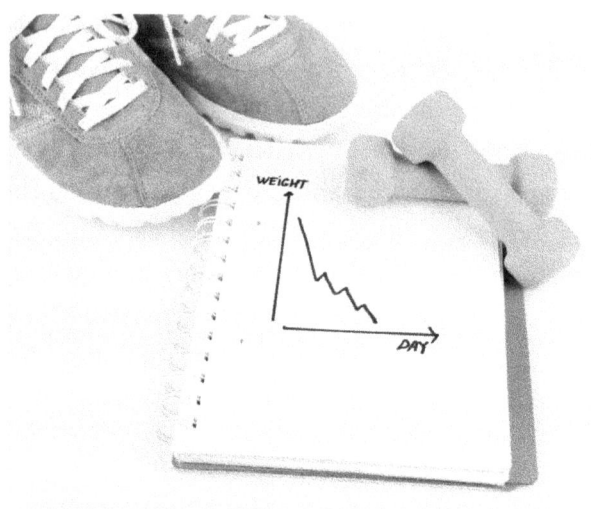

Be aware of how you are changing for the better. It shows hard work paying off and encourages you to continue to change for the better.

A very important thing for you to do when you are on a fitness program is to track how you are progressing. This will keep you highly motivated, especially when you see that you are becoming what you set out to be.

Weigh yourself regularly but don't obsess about weight. Weight loss will taper off and come in small increments. You may have weeks when you lose nothing. Don't freak out, this is not uncommon. What is more important is how you feel? How do you look in clothes? How many inches have you lost? These items are just as important as a number on a scale.

If you run keep track of distance and time. When you are working out keep track of weight and reps. Tracking your heart rate, blood sugar level, blood pressure? Keep monitoring it and write it down. Write it all down!

We as humans are very result-oriented people. We want to see facts and figures. We want to see things as raw as they can be. This is the reason why tracking your progress continuously will help you immensely.

When you see that your waist size has come down from 38" to 36", when you see that you can get into skimpier shorts, when you see that you are closer to touching your toes than before, you become pleased with yourself. You see that your efforts are paying off. This keeps the fire burning within you.

Get use to looking at yourself in mirrors. People who are overweight are typically ashamed of their bodies and try to conceal them from themselves and everyone else. This is no longer the case for you. When working out watch yourself in the mirrors. Watch your form and watch your muscles expand and contract. Look at yourself clothed and naked. Take pride in your new body, learn to love it and appreciate it. When you love your body you will have more love in your heart. Take pride on your accomplishments and determination but stay focused on where you are going.

So keep looking as much as you want. It is only when you are in love with your body that you will respect it and honor it. No one will love your body more than you so don't be shy and don't be embarrassed. Look at it, love it and be proud of yourself!

Chapter 8: Stay Motivated with Incentives

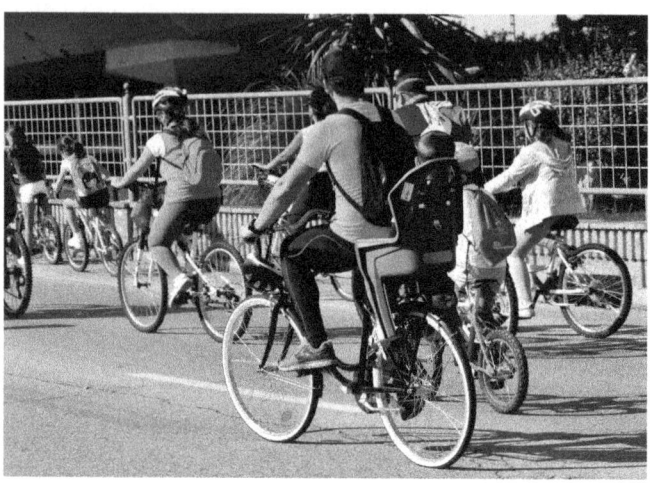

Rewarding yourself is one of the best ways to ensure that you keep doing the right things.

Time and again, reward yourself for your achievements. However, don't reward yourself with a food. This more than likely will be a habit you will have to be aware of and break. As a society we are fixated on food. When we are happy, the first thing that comes to our mind is a treat that involves the worst kinds of unhealthy foods possible. And this is what brings on most of the health problems that we face today. We could do much better from a health point of view if we cured our fixation with food.

Instead, give yourself a healthy incentive. Go on a trip, update your wardrobe, treat yourself to a spa day, etc. Reward yourself with something you want or want to do. Maybe something you would have never have dreamed of doing when you were heavier due to physical limitations or just being embarrassed by your size.

However, one of the best incentives is looking in the mirror. When you see the improved shape you are in, that is a reward in itself. Take photos of yourself throughout your journey. Keep these photos available for comparison. Congratulate yourself on obstacles you have overcome to obtain your current body. The photos will remind you of where you started, how far you have come, and that your end goal is obtainable and within your reach.

Shopping for new clothes is fun and very motivating. Buy clothes that fit your newly reworked body. Fitting into smaller sizes is the proof of your hard work and should bring a sense of achievement.

You should understand that when you measure or weigh yourself at home and see that you have reduced, you are happy. But when you are able to buy a brand of jeans you couldn't previously fit into or you can buy a less restrictive and more comfortable smaller bra you see the practical connotations of your health and fitness program. You actually see the benefits. This will motivate you to keep working towards your goal. The benefits are proof that your discipline and hard work has produced results and is worth it.

Chapter 9: Make the Effort – Exercise Even if You Don't Feel Like It

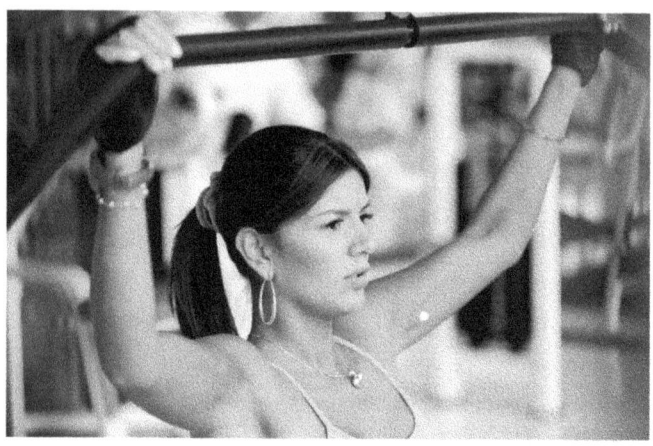

Get yourself to the gym each day, even if you don't think you want to work out. Just heading out to the gym can help you immensely.

One of the ways in which you can motivate to keep working out is by simply making the effort to go to the gym. Research shows that most people who quit their gyms don't do it because exercising is too hard; they do quit because they don't want to make the trip to the gym! Sounds silly, but it is true. If you have joined a gym before, you will be aware of this feeling. You don't mind the workouts, but you loathe getting dressed to exercise and physically going to the gym, which may be early in the morning cutting into your sleep.

If you don't want to go to the gym on one particular day, remember this. Tell yourself that you will just warm up a bit on the treadmill and then leave. Tell yourself that you won't do anything that needs you to exert much. When you convince yourself of this, you are likelier to head to the gym.

But when you are there, you will see a change happening in your way of thinking. When you see all those people diligently working out, you too will become motivated. And when you start out on the treadmill, you will find that your stamina is building. When that happens, you will tell yourself that you could try one more exercise. You might go on to the exercise bike. That may induce you to go to the weights and then the resistance training and so on. Sooner than you think, you will find that you have completed your workout!

Studies show that this approach works in ninety percent of the cases i.e. ninety percent of the people who come to the gym reluctantly, thinking that they will only work out for five minutes, end up working out their full routine.

The same applies with other things. If you are feeling lazy about going for jogging, convince yourself by saying that you will walk briskly. You might tell yourself that you would do nothing more than stretch and one lap around the park. But once you are there you become motivated and do more than what you initially intended.

Chapter 10: You Can Do It! Sticking to Your Health and Fitness Goals

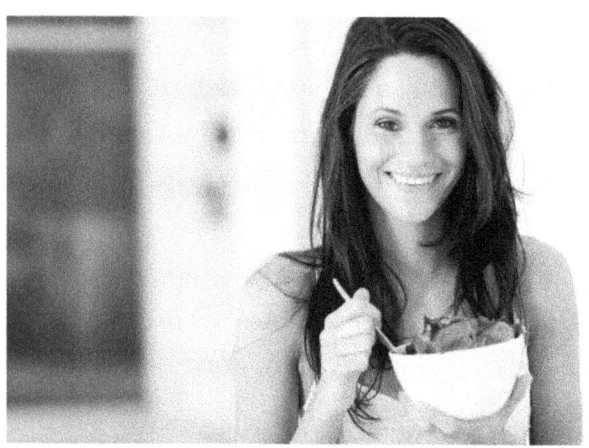

You can keep going, just be convinced that you can.

Given the large rate of failure of health and fitness program worldwide, it is easy to see why anyone will have a fair share of apprehension when they think about making healthy lifestyle changes. They are bound to wonder whether making healthy changes will work for them or not. Even when you join a gym, however enthusiastic you are, somewhere in the corner of your mind you wonder how long you will stick to the routine. These thoughts are damaging when you haven't even had your first workout at the gym.

You need to condition your mind into thinking positively about the program you are about to join. Don't keep any space for pessimism. There is no reason why you should think that your health goals won't work for you. Think that it will work. Think about all the benefits you will get from the up and coming changes.

Envision a sexier body, a healthier heart, improved physical capacity, shopping for smaller clothes and you will want to follow through with your goals.

Think about how you will become a better individual inside and outside. Think about how you will be able to do things you want to do because your health won't restrict you. Think about how your bank balance will improve because you will become more productive. Think about how you your confidence will improve as well as your personal relationships.

You will be able to spend more quality time with your friends and family. You will no longer sit on the sidelines embarrassed by your physical limitations or body image. You will be able to join the fun. If nothing else, take a look at your children, if you have them. Wouldn't you like to set a positive example for them?

We now come back full circle to motivation and determination. The best way to make lifestyle changes stick is write down goals, be determined on achieving those goals and to stay motivated. You have to stay focused and not let small set-backs and failures throw you completely of your course. Celebrate small successes and build from the them. Remember the bigger picture which is your end goal which is ultimately a fitter, healthier, and happy you.

CHAPTER 11: HEALTH AND FITNESS AFFIRMATIONS

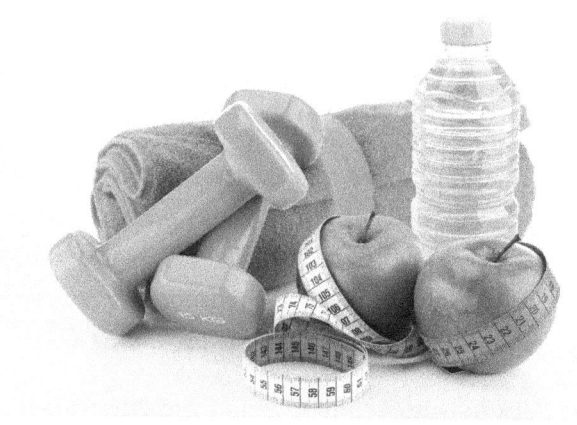

What Affirmations Are and How to Use Them

Affirmations are self-talk statements presented to the subconscious. These fresh images are viewed as "credible" by the subconscious and are placed in the area of subconscious having to do with the power to enhance the ability to pull up particular powerful memories with less work. Through this special imagery a person can develop the inner tools for the correct mindset for achieving anything they want to do, enhance, or change.

Why Do We Need Affirmations?

Oftentimes individuals believe good and beneficial self-talk memories are a false belief and don't exist, but the subconscious recognizes where they're located and will pull them out when needed.

These forms of affirmations make fresh neural tracts in the mind, enhancing the ability to "see" these fresh powerful images. Stale images related to negativity, weaknesses, deficiency of initiative, frail goal images are decreased. When the mind discovers new affirmations the subconscious sees them as "tangible."

You've likely observed a common element in those who are successful in business and in life. These winners and successful individuals tend to be enthusiastic and zealous, in all aspects of their lives. This exuberance can be infectious, and it tends to rub off on all those persons around them. A positive attitude and the determination to turn that attitude into results are crucial to success for anything you do in business and in life.

You see, a positive attitude is a valuable asset, no matter what you are trying to do. You really ought to assume the habit of doing regular positive affirmations. Making positive affirmations a part of your daily function is a great way to alter your thoughts and help you reach goals.

It's never too early or too late to begin this cycle of positive affirmations, and even those just beginning down a new road may benefit from a positive attitude. Even if the thing you're trying to accomplish seems insignificant it's crucial to display a positive attitude, and not let negativity sneak in to steal your thunder.

Affirmations are Fantastic - But They Have to be Used Correctly

Self-affirmations are positive statements or self-scripts that might condition the subconscious so that you're able to develop a more positive perception of yourself. Affirmations might help you to change adverse behaviors or achieve the correct mindset, and they can likewise help undo the harm caused by negative scripts, those things which we repeatedly tell ourselves (or which others repeatedly tell us) that add to a negative self-perception and affect our success.

Read through the following affirmations and write down those that speak to you. Put them on a 3x5 index card for convenience. Repeat the affirmations on a daily basis's at least once a day. Say the affirmations out loud and with conviction.

I AM living a long and healthy life.

I always contribute in healthy ways to my body.

I eat healthy, nutritious and digestible food every day.

God gave me a healthy body and in gratitude, I take Good care of myself.

My strong body has fully recovered and healed.

I drink large amounts of thirst quenching water every day.

I have a healthy spirit, mind and body.

I love myself and I am perfectly healthy.

I accept healthy eating as a way of life.

Working out improves my mood.

Finding time for exercise is becoming easier and more natural.

I change my life by transforming myself.

I am full of energy and vitality and my mind is calm and peaceful.

I look wonderful.

I am getting stronger every day.

I am flexible because I exercise.

I have a strong desire to be healthy and strong

My fitness routine is interesting and varied.

Sleep is sacred. I show my love for my body by giving it the rest it needs. I sleep deeply.

I choose to change my eating habits and I successfully do so.

I ignore false messages of hunger and eat only when necessary.

I always train with intensity.

I live a healthy lifestyle.

I am dedicated to improving my fitness. I am focused on achieving a high level of fitness.

I maintain a healthy weight.

I am stronger because I exercise.

I take good care of myself.

I am healthy and energetic.

I am intelligent and sexy.

I am physically fit.

Living an active lifestyle is just what I do.

I am fit, healthy and attractive.

I love and appreciate my body.

I love to exercise.

I am fit and healthy.

Other people will look to me for fitness inspiration.

I will increase my endurance.

My appearance will improve along with my fitness level.

Every day in every way I am getting healthier and healthier and feeling better and better.

I avoid junk food. I eat healthy, nutritious food that benefits my body and large quantity of water that cleanses my body.

I think only positive thoughts and am always happy and joyous, no matter what the external conditions are.

I can eat right without hurting anyone's feelings.

I exchange high fat foods for high energy foods and all excess fat is now being removed from me.

I let go of all reasons and excuses for not eating healthy meals.

Fresh vegetables feel and taste good in my mouth.

I will continue to reach my fitness goals.

I push myself to the max.

I am losing two pounds each week.

I always feel good. As a result, my body feels good and I radiate good feelings.

I willingly keep my meal portions small.

I am burning fat when I do aerobic exercises.

The Universe provides more than enough food for me.

I am fit and active.

I am accomplishing great feats every day.

I will create 30 minutes in my schedule to exercise each day.

Every day in every way I am becoming fitter and healthier.

I get all the vitamins and nutrients I need.

I enjoy my daily workouts and they make me feel energetic.

I am energetic.

I choose fruits and vegetables over salty, sugary high fat foods every time.

I am beautiful.

I am happy with the way exercise makes me look and feel.

Good health is my birth right. I bless my body daily and take good care of it.

I am extremely fit.

I have reached my weight loss goals.

I choose to work out every day for a beautiful body.

My daily exercises make me stronger and fitter.

I am of a strong heart and steel body. I am vigorous, energetic and full of vitality.

My stamina is high.

I successfully release the desire to eat beyond the point of being full.

I like the way exercise makes me feel.

Every passing day my body becomes more energetic, more healthy.

I will be the strongest and healthiest I can possibly be.

I can do it.

Every day is a new day full of hope, happiness and health.

I am slender.

I listen to my body and pay attention to what it is telling me.

The adrenalin rush of a hard workout exhilarates me.

I like to workout.

I love life and I am immune to the temptation of eating processed foods.

I eat the right foods at the right times.

Working towards my fitness goals is a priority in my life.

I am healthy and sexy.

I easily replace foods containing refined sugar with natural foods.

I enjoy my workouts.

I create my own beauty. I take care of my body, outside and in. I feel and look my best.

Others see me as someone who is extremely fit and healthy.

I am a healthy and fit man/woman.

I treat my body as a temple. It is holy, it is clean and it is full of goodness.

I am taking my exercise to the next level.

I am strong and can handle anything that challenges me today.

I breathe deeply, exercise regularly and feed only good nutritious food to my body.

I am exercising for an extra 15 minutes today.

I am allowed to decline food and do so in total peace.

I am adding weights to my work out routine.

I am free of diabetes, free of blood pressure problems and free of all life threatening diseases.

My workout is something I look forward to.

I am excited to exercise.

Perfect health is my divine right, and I claim it now.

I refuse to let other people influence me to eat too much.

I can feel the fat burning when I jog.

I forgive myself for eating the wrong foods and I transcend all feelings of unworthiness.

I only eat the foods that are good for me.

I can easily pump myself up and get in the right frame of mind.

Eating right is easy and fun for me. I love my body and take good care of it by eating correctly.

I am full of energy.

Being dedicated to a regular fitness routine is easy for me.

I release the need for foods that cause indigestion and discomfort.

Being physically fit is the foundation for a happy and healthy life.

I substitute high fat foods with high water content foods.

I am becoming more physically fit.

I love fitness training.

For me, eating and emotional comfort are separate and I forgive myself for overeating.

My body will grow stronger.

I will eat healthier and continue to exercise.

I replace dieting with healthy eating principles and habits.

I will become quicker and have faster reflexes.

My metabolism has improved as a result of my exercises and I am leaner and fitter.

Healthy eating and I are one and I am richly rewarded for my healthy eating habits.

MEET THE AUTHOR

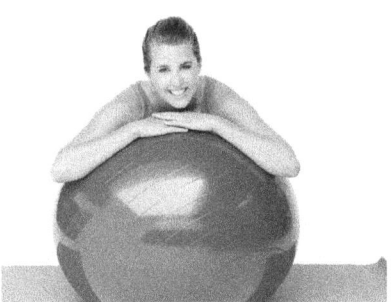

Certified personal trainer, nutrition and diet specialist and a wellness coach Kelly Larson's goal is to give as many people as possible the tools to start living a healthier lifestyle.

Kelly believes that every person can achieve the body of their dreams through fitness, healthy eating and a balanced lifestyle. Kelly follows her own personal health and fitness philosophies and believes that a "perfect body" is not a realistic goal. The importance of good health should drive and motivate people to achieve better fitness and a better body. When you take care of your body as a whole you will start to feel better and your body will transform into looking better.

Kelly lives in sunny Florida and enjoys spending time with family and friends. Kelly is passionate about music, scuba diving and new adventures. In her spare time, Kelly volunteers at her local animal shelter.

MORE BOOKS BY KELLY LARSON

Green Tea for Weight Loss and Health: Detox, Boost Immunity, Lower Cholesterol, Increase Metabolism, Burn Calories

Nutritional Prevention and Cures for Better Health: Natural Alternatives to Restore Your Health

Six Pack Abs: How to Get Ripped Abs: The Truth on How to Reveal Your Six Pack Abs With Diet and Exercise

Stop Dieting and Lose Weight: The Ultimate Manual on Losing Weight, Getting Healthy and Changing Your Mindset about Food and Diets

The Ultimate Manual on Losing Weight, Getting Healthy and Changing Your Mindset about Food and Diets: The Ultimate Guide to a Hot Summer Body

www.ingramcontent.com/pod-product-compliance
Ingram Content Group UK Ltd.
Pitfield, Milton Keynes, MK11 3LW, UK
UKHW022218230426
12048UKWH00016BA/916